D.I.V.E.R.S.I.T.Y.

D.I.V.E.R.S.I.T.Y.

A Guide to Working with Diversity
and Developing Cultural Sensitivity

Vivian Okeze-Tirado

Jessica Kingsley Publishers
London and Philadelphia

First published in Great Britain in 2021 by VOT Training,
West Sussex, UK as Diversity Acrostic Poem
This edition published in Great Britain in 2023 by Jessica Kingsley Publishers
An imprint of Hodder & Stoughton Ltd
An Hachette UK Company

1

Front cover image source: Timi Phillips (@artby_timi).

A CIP catalogue record for this title is available from the British Library
and the Library of Congress

ISBN 978 1 83997 631 5
eISBN 978 1 83997 632 2

Printed and bound in Great Britain by TJ Books Ltd

Jessica Kingsley Publishers' policy is to use papers that are natural, renewable
and recyclable products and made from wood grown in sustainable forests.
The logging and manufacturing processes are expected to conform to the
environmental regulations of the country of origin.

Jessica Kingsley Publishers
Carmelite House
50 Victoria Embankment
London EC4Y 0DZ

www.jkp.com

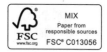

MIX
Paper from
responsible sources
FSC® C013056

Diversity is the norm in nature.
Being part of a minority is being part of the whole.

CONTENTS

PROLOGUE

The murder in broad daylight of an unarmed black man, George Floyd, in the United States in May 2020, stirred me to put everything aside to complete this book.

This book is based on the Diversity Acrostic Poem I created in 2015. An acrostic poem is one in which the letters of each line spell out a word, name, or phrase when read vertically.

I created this poem by utilizing the word 'diversity' and reproducing phrases that best describe the act of working with difference and becoming a culturally sensitive practitioner. This book essentially is structured around the poem and supports individuals and professionals to be culturally sensitive.

Through this book, my intention is to advocate for justice and equality, anti-oppressive and anti-discriminatory practice, and the embracing of diversity and inclusion in our society. I will focus on cultural difference and anti-racist practice, reflecting the tense racial climate at the time of writing in 2020 and the prominence of the Black Lives Matter movement.

Over the years, there have been arguments by scholars that education in the western world and government policies and regulations continue to perpetuate white supremacy (Ugwuegbula 2020). As Katherine Kallehauge, Junior Editor of the Education and Equal Rights Society, says:

> There is a divide in education, a subtle colour line, which veils the legacy of white, European powers and their relations to the non-white others. Not only has the veil kept non-whiteness at bay and rejected access to knowledge, it has distorted white heritage of violence against the peoples within Africa and those in diaspora, enduring the enforcement of racial inequality and supremacy. (Kallehauge 2021)

Further, this societal trend has become entrenched for generations, with white members of society becoming accustomed to privileges not afforded to minoritized groups.

This way of living remains extremely advantageous to the privileged group, while hugely disadvantageous to the minoritized groups. Shifting such an entrenched culture will require a monumental force, cutting from the very top to the bottom, and is bound to generate continuous fierce resistance by those accustomed to the privilege.

In recent years, there have been questions around whether universal education and training across secondary and tertiary institutions places adequate emphasis on anti-discriminatory and anti-oppressive practice. This is particularly the case in humanitarian professions such as my own discipline of social work, which purport to promote social change and social justice.

In July 2020, the Chief Social Worker for Children and Families in England, Isabelle Trowler, wrote to the Chief Executive of Social Work England, the regulatory body, urging him to address 'serious concerns' from students over a lack of focus on anti-discriminatory practice.

Universities are being called on to embed teaching on white privilege and fragility in anti-racist training. This is encouraging, but it remains to be seen how this will be achieved.

About the author

This book is all about people, how we relate to one another and understanding our different perspectives, so it makes sense for me to introduce myself at the start.

My name is Vivian Obiageli Okeze-Tirado. I am a black African born in Nigeria to Engineer (DR) Mathias Okeze and Mrs Mercy Okeze, from Ibusa and Okwe in Delta State,

Nigeria. I am nationalized as Irish. I am a wife and mother to two children. My husband, veterinary surgeon Francisco Tirado, is white Spanish, and our daughter Salome and son Lorenzo were born in Ireland and are both Irish by nationality. I am the first of five sisters, Josephine, Anastasia, Theresa, Cynthia, and a brother, Victor.

I am the Equality, Diversity and Inclusion Lead for West Sussex County Council Children Services, and a social work practice educator. My first degree was a BA Hons in Linguistics, followed by a Master's degree in Business Administration and Management. Prior to entering social work, I was a business banking officer.

I decided to move into social work to pursue a more humanitarian career around improving the outcomes for vulnerable children and families.

I obtained my second Master's degree in Social Work from Brighton University in 2014. I also obtained an MA in Advanced Professional Practice: Practice Education Combined at the University of Chichester in 2018. As a practice educator, I have enjoyed facilitating trainings for foster carers, social workers and management staff, both within and outside West Sussex and including universities and fostering agencies.

I have always been keen on social work research and practice development to enhance the experiences of children, families and professionals from all backgrounds. I am passionate about promoting diversity, equality and inclusion and I enjoy developing ideas, materials and strategies to enhance personal and professional practice.

I have championed diversity/anti-racist practice/cultural competence workshops both within and outside West Sussex Children Services.

In 2021, I was named social justice advocate and social worker of the year at the Social Worker of the Year Awards for my work in creating diversity workshops for foster carers and social work colleagues following George Floyd's murder.

I was privileged to present my diversity model at the annual Joint Social Work Education and Research Conference (JSWEC) UK at the Leeds Beckett University in June 2022.

I advocate strongly for equality, diversity and inclusion because I believe we live in a diverse world of people with varied talents, each contributing to a thriving economy. Failing to acknowledge, respect or avail ourselves of the benefits of this is nothing but tragic.

What is this book, and who is it for?

D.I.V.E.R.S.I.T.Y. is designed as an educational resource written for individuals and professionals who are seeking knowledge on how to work effectively with diversity and become culturally competent.

It is intended to be an accessible and easy-to-use practice tool for social workers, healthcare staff, teachers, counsellors, university lecturers and all those involved in people-facing professions. Other readers might include public servants who directly engage with the individuals and communities and who need to communicate with understanding and empathy.

Throughout the book, I'll often use the term 'helping professionals' to keep things simple and avoid repetition.

It's a simple idea, which can be adapted to many different settings. The book can be used:

- individually for your own practice, to encourage discourse within teams or groups, or with clients
- to create a reflective discourse with clients young or old
- to support students in secondary, college and university education.

A chance to reflect

At the end of each chapter, there is a section called 'Reflection notes' with lines for you to fill in – to reflect on each theme, and to relate it to your daily work. The book is intended to prompt not just thoughts but changes in habits, attitudes and actions!

Through reflection, you will be able to identify barriers to working with diversity and promoting justice and equality. To promote societal growth, social change and social justice, members of a society need to acknowledge and respect diversity while recognizing and challenging oppression and discrimination in their day-to-day life, work and actions.

The premise is that racism is entrenched in our society, be it conscious, unconscious or institutional. Therefore, it is only logical that in trying to combat it, we must look at it from the perspective of how it impacts institutional learning.

Bearing in mind that readers may be busy individuals and professionals, I have made this book concise and to the point.

Each letter of D.I.V.E.R.S.I.T.Y. in the acrostic poem represents a chapter of the book. One letter of the poem includes personal anecdotes and humour – I hope readers will find it amusing, yet educational.

The book begins with an open letter to all, which pays tribute to George Floyd and which was published in England by *West Sussex County Times* in June 2020. As a human being and a social work practitioner living through these tense racial times, I did not want to sit back and do nothing because that would not be right. It is often said that success is not only what you accomplish but what you can motivate others to do. I hope that this book will serve as a practical tool to awaken racial consciousness and arouse empathy for the plight of black and ethnic minority groups in a world where white privilege is not only perceptible but overpowering.

Why this is important: diversity, equality and the law

Promoting diversity is not only a moral imperative, but also a legal one, and is embedded within professional frameworks for many helping practitioners.

I write as a social worker based in England, where professionals are expected to have an understanding of equality law – this book will help you to undertake systematic self-analysis and to test your understanding of these attributes.

However, the core principles of equality and diversity which lie at the heart of this book are embedded in legislation internationally, so wherever you are based, you can apply this tool to the legal framework in which you are working.

Here are some examples:

- UK Equality Act 2010
- US Equality Act 2021, which expands on the 1964 Civil Rights Act
- Australian federal anti-discrimination laws of 1991

- Canadian Human Rights Act of 1977, which covers the equality acts in the federal jurisdictions, while each province has its own human rights.

My hope

I'll leave you with my hope: that this book: *D.I.V.E.R.S.I.T.Y.: A Guide to Working with Diversity and Developing Cultural Sensitivity* encourages you to connect to the plight of the less privileged in our society and make a difference.

George Floyd: A call for Justice and Equality – an open letter to all...

by Vivian Okeze-Tirado (first published in the West Sussex County Times *18 June, 2020)*

Dear all,

I hope this letter meets you all well. I would like to lend my voice concerning the gruesome murder in broad daylight of a fellow human being, an unarmed black man George Floyd in the US seen as an act of racism all around the world. This event affects us all because it is a painful wound to humanity. The video, as widely shown, is quite distressing and saddening to watch. No human being should have to undergo such treatment regardless of their race, colour, religion, sex, etc... Such display of racial injustice and inequality is not an isolated incident but has been ongoing for decades, not just in the US but all over the western world/Europe, etc. A systematic degradation, covert and overt discrimination, plundering, limitation, restrictions, etc.

To those who think that the recent anti-racism protests have gone on long enough, the question is; what is being done or proposed by the leaders in terms of reforms and policies to create real, lasting change around this issue? Racism cannot continue to be ignored. Folks standing aside or assuming ignorance is no longer an option. We can now see that the three police officers who stood by, watched, and did nothing during the murder of George Floyd are now facing charges of accomplices to murder. This is what happens when we stand by and do nothing amid oppression and injustice – a lesson to be learnt by all.

To those who say that George Floyd was a 'criminal', what happened to 'innocent until proven guilty'? Are criminals now meant to be killed gruesomely on the streets by law enforcement agents? Also, is there any human being who can testify to doing no wrong in their lifetime? Whatever that wrong would have looked like! People have a right to turn their life around without prejudice or judgement or people digging up their past at the slightest provocation, particularly when they are of a certain race.

The worldwide protests and mixed protesters from all walks of life, all cultures, all colours, etc..., all around the world, show that there is hope yet. It means that there are humanitarian people out there who can recognize injustice, show love and solidarity to one another, and even risk their lives doing so for justice and equality. There is hope yet...

Where does hope lie...?

The ball is now in the court of our leaders, powerful individuals and groups to create positive change once and for all. No more hypocrisy, no more distraction tactics or lip service, no more political correctness, or well-drafted diplomatic speeches. Enough is enough. We are all involved. We are all connected; we need each other; let us refrain from feeling threatened and embrace diversity with all positivity.

If you ever need to know how connected we all are, please refer to the recent Covid-19 pandemic, which effectively spread rapidly from country to country, person to person regardless of class, race, gender, colour, rich, poor, powerful, or non-powerful.

If you are still feeling detached about the plight of Black & Ethnic minority groups and Black Lives Matter movement, please go and watch the film *The Boy in the Striped Pyjamas*, based on the novel by John Boyne (2006). In this film, we see how the son of a Nazi commander became, by default, a victim of the gassing of the Jews in concentration camps because of his friendship with a Jewish child at the time.

D.I.V.E.R.S.I.T.Y.

As we know, children have no prejudices except what they have been taught. Unknown to the commander, his son would become a victim of his heartless orders to gas the Jews in one of the concentration camps. Although this film is based on fiction, it does indeed show how social connectedness could lead to events that we, as individuals, have no control over, especially with the growing young generation beginning to see the truth and working in unity, friendship and solidarity.

We are all indeed connected...

Let us care enough to connect

Connect to the plight of the disadvantaged people,

There is room for all in our society

Let us be bold and courageous and stand up for equality

Stand up for justice and fair play in all nations

#There is unity in diversity#

#There is power in diversity#

#There is growth in diversity#

#Black lives matter#

#We know all lives matter#

#Help is needed with Black Lives Matter so that black lives can matter too#

#Rise up above colour#

#Rise up and show love#

#Rise up for justice and equality#

It is the right thing to do. Now is the time...

To George Floyd and others killed unjustly on account of the colour of their skin... Rest in peace.

EQUALITY AND DIVERSITY

What is equality?

'Equality is the right of different groups of people to have a similar social position and receive the same treatment.' (Cambridge English Dictionary)

'Equality is the right of different groups of people to receive the same treatment.' (Oxford American Dictionary)

Equality is underpinned by legal frameworks that place statutory duty on individuals, communities and organizations to ensure that no one under the protected characteristics is disadvantaged.

The equality protected characteristics in most countries of the world include the multi-dimensional layers of diversity, including age, disability, gender, race, religion or belief and marriage.

The US Equality Act was passed by Congress in March 2021, expanding on the 1964 Civil Rights Act, and includes protection against discrimination based on sexual orientation and gender identity.

Similarly, in Australia, the federal anti-discrimination law of 1991 is contained in legislations such as the Age Discrimination Act of 2004, the Disability Discrimination Act of 1992, the Racial Discrimination Act of 1975 and the Sex Discrimination Act of 1984.

In simplistic terms, 'equality' means that all individuals should be treated equally, and should have an equal chance to experience day-to-day life, work, and opportunities as others, regardless of any of the characteristics mentioned above.

In other words, equality ensures that diversity is acknowledged and respected.

Organizations and government departments at all levels have a moral as well as a legal duty to consider the equality protected attributes and ensure that every person can fulfil their potential at work, regardless of protected characteristics.

'Every person, regardless of their ethnicity or background, should be able to fulfil their potentials at work. That is the business case as well as the moral case.' (McGregor-Smith Review 2017)

What is diversity?

Diversity – 'The fact of many different types of things or people being included in something; a range of different things or people.' (Cambridge English Dictionary)

'The condition or fact of being different or varied; variety.' (Oxford American Dictionary)

Diversity means the difference in people, behaviour, culture, language, religion or beliefs. The terms 'diversity' and 'equality' are often used together.

A global movement

For me, as a social worker based in England, 'diversity' forms one of the nine professional capabilities adopted by the

British Association of Social Workers (BASW) in 2018. The Professional Capabilities Framework is designed to help social workers practice more efficiently. It stipulates that 'Social Workers must recognise diversity and apply anti-discriminatory and anti-oppressive principles in practice' (British Association of Social Workers 2018).

Social Work England Professional Standards stipulate: 'Social workers must promote the rights, strengths, and wellbeing of people, families, and communities...' They should, 'recognise differences across diverse communities and challenge the impact of disadvantage and discrimination on people and their families and communities' (standard 1.5) and 'promote social justice, helping to confront and resolve issues of inequality and inclusion' (standard 1.6).

Do you know how diversity and equality relate to your own professional code or standards? If not, find out!

On its website, the United States Department of Labor states: 'By fostering a culture of diversity – or a capacity to appreciate and value individual differences – employers benefit from varied perspectives on how to confront business challenges and achieve success.'

On his first day in office in 2021, US President Joe Biden signed an executive order to advance racial equity and support 'underserved communities'. He acknowledged the benefits of diversity, the skills and talents it brings to the table, together with high workplace performance and productivity.

He also acknowledged that advancing equity, civil rights and racial injustice was a whole government responsibility. Joe Biden's words and actions showed a level of insight into arguably one of the most potent and prevalent subject matters in the history of the nation.

Jacinda Ardern, Prime Minister of New Zealand, one of the most thriving nations in the world, stated in her speech in March 2019 in the wake of Christchurch terrorist attack: 'We don't let racism exist because racism breeds extremism... Let New Zealand be a place where there is no tolerance for racism ever and that's something we can all do' (Ardern 2019).

She also stated in her UN Speech, also in March 2019, 'If I could distil down to one concept that we are pursuing in New Zealand, it is simple and it is this: kindness.'

These statements indicate a leader who not only appreciates diversity but is also keen to promote emotional and cultural sensitivity, key ingredients that form a humane, fair and just society.

In the recent past, the Australian Government Department of Health produced action plans to support inclusive and diverse workplaces such as the Reconciliation Action Plan

(RAP), outlining how the government proposes to work with Aboriginal people and Torres Strait Islanders to build a stable relationship and increase their life chances and opportunities. Part of the focus of its diversity and inclusion strategy 2019–2022 is on cultural and linguistic diversity, gender diversity and equality.

These are all very positive ideologies; however, the challenge lies with achieving the reality.

We live in a multicultural world; diversity exists all around us. The ability to acknowledge this and interact or work well with it is an absolute necessity. This means that individuals and professionals not only need to be skilled up but also seek ways in which to challenge acts of discrimination and oppression around them. A good understanding of the individual self and privilege is key in forming and managing personal and professional relationships with members of a diverse world.

WHAT IS CULTURAL COMPETENCE?

Cultural competence in social work 'entails understanding the cultural differences of people in need of social services. Social workers who demonstrate cultural competence strive to understand the cultures of the people they serve and approach them with cultural sensitivity and respect'. (Virginia Commonwealth University 2019)

Although this definition from the Virginia Commonwealth University relates to the social work profession, it could equally be applied to related professions. Cultural competence is simply the ability to appreciate and interact effectively with people from various cultural backgrounds. One of the best ways to grow your confidence and cultural competence is to learn about other cultures. Becoming culturally competent is a key skill to have in the 21st century. It is a skill that evolves, meaning that you continue to develop over time. The learning in this area never ends and the social skills and behaviours you acquire will enable you to *work well* with diversity, not just tolerate it. If you are in the privileged group, you can learn to support the less privileged or those in the disadvantaged group to reach their full potential by acknowledging and respecting their experiences and perspectives – building and reinforcing understanding and relationships.

Professionals don't necessarily have to be experts, but it does help if you have a keenness to acquire new knowledge and a willingness to apply it in your work.

For example, for a social worker in children's services, a child or young person's cultural heritage and identity cannot be overlooked. It should be at the forefront of practice.

This is the same for a teacher imparting knowledge to children from diverse backgrounds at school.

Psychologists or therapists should seek to first understand their client's culture before proffering advice or healing.

Cultural sensitivity is demanded in all areas of practice, in education, social care, social work, healthcare and any area of public service. The need for cultural responsiveness has become amplified and widely advocated in the wake of the murder of George Floyd.

There have of course been many more killings reported in the states of America since George Floyd. In May 2022, in Buffalo, New York, just weeks short of the anniversary of the murder of George Floyd, an 18-year-old white boy, Payton S. Gendron, opened fire on black people in a supermarket, leaving ten people dead and three wounded. The young shooter was arrested and taken into custody.

My question is, if the case were reversed and it was a black man shooting at white people in a supermarket, wearing a bulletproof jacket or not, would he have left that mall alive or been allowed to surrender? Let us reflect on that for a minute... I am sure you will agree with me that the answer is a capital NO. I would call this a prime example of the back-and-forth of racism and white privilege birthed by white supremacy. No wonder President Joe Biden in his response to the event, stated: 'White supremacy is a poison running through our body politics' (Helmore & Smith 2022).

Post George Floyd, it is clear that some government agencies and organizations are slowly beginning to make subtle changes. They have begun to formulate policies and put some actions in place to address marginalization and non-representation. Roles are being created and professionals recruited as accountable persons for equality, diversity and inclusion. This shows that there is some systemic recognition of a problem and an attempt to remedy it.

At the risk of stating the obvious, diversity is crucial for societal growth. Society not taking advantage of the benefits is a tragedy. Individuals or professionals can no longer shy away or pretend that the subject matter does not involve them. There is an individual and collective responsibility, hence working effectively with diversity is fundamental and critical.

Tragic events like the Buffalo shooting are ongoing, particularly in the US. It is no longer news that black Americans are three times more likely to be killed by the police, despite being the considerable minority in the population (Aljazeera News 2021).

In December 2021, the case of Child Q made headline news and caused huge uproar in the UK regarding the discriminatory treatment of a 15-year-old strip searched on biased suspicion of her possessing cannabis. The search was reportedly requested by her school despite her being on her period. Needless to say, no drugs were found on her.

According to the Guardian news website (2022) sadly,

> A recent freedom of information request to the Met revealed that the force conducted about 9,000 strip searches on children in the past five years. In Hackney Borough of England,

where child Q is from, 60% of the children strip-searched last year were black.

Why cultural competence matters

More awareness and attention have been created around racial inequality in our society in the months and years following these tragic events. More and more professionals, government officials and politicians should pay proper attention and discuss cultural competence.

Ignorance should no longer be an excuse. In late 2020, some months after the murder of George Floyd, the news and social media in the UK revealed that a prominent public figure, Football Association Chairman Greg Clarke, was forced to resign from his position after referring to black footballers as 'coloured'. He used outdated and inappropriate terminology while addressing British MPs in Parliament.

Unfortunately for him, he paid a huge price for the improper use of language, especially in the tense racial climate of the very extraordinary and noteworthy year of 2020 – a year that one could safely refer to as the year of George Floyd.

It would seem that basic knowledge of appropriate terminology is not common within the Football Association, even though it is richly endowed with players from diverse backgrounds.

Many more professionals will fall victim to the consequences of using inappropriate language, but among helping professionals, where relationships and sensitivity are such an important area of our work, practitioners can't afford to lack cultural competence.

In the social work profession, the importance of cultural competence cannot be over-emphasized both in children's services and adult services. Recent years have seen the influx of children into care from various cultural backgrounds, with parents from different cultures. Social workers must promote the identities of all vulnerable children, as it is crucial for building their self-esteem.

One of the core values of social work is the pursuit of social justice and anti-oppressive and anti-discriminatory practice. Social workers cannot claim to effectively embed this principle without acknowledging and respecting diversity, and promoting inclusion and integration in society.

Most of the service users we work with in social care, particularly children and young people, come from diverse backgrounds, with different cultures, experiences, worldviews and so on.

In my view, social work is a career like no other, a purely humanitarian service to society's most vulnerable members.

Because you're reading this book, I imagine that you are like me – a professional who takes pride in thinking of yourself as a change-maker in society. To make real change, we must strive to work genuinely and effectively with diversity – otherwise, it will be impossible to create the very difference that we wish to make.

At this point, you may be wondering what cultural sensitivity looks like in the most practical terms.

Well, let's look at this straightforward and easy-to-understand concept – the Diversity Acrostic Poem.

D Decide to be a culturally sensitive practitioner

I Invite people to talk about their cultures, values, beliefs and experiences

V Value service users' history, individuality and differences

E Explore clients' realities and show curiosity

R Reflect on the information and knowledge received

S Scrutinize yourself – personal SWOT analysis (strengths, weaknesses, opportunities, threats)

I Identify strategies to aid your work

T Train yourself to treat people, children and families individually

Y Yield to culturally sensitive practice

Decide to be a Culturally Sensitive Practitioner

Working effectively with diversity and becoming a culturally competent practitioner is a fundamental requirement for becoming a proficient worker within the helping professions. You must decide the kind of worker you wish to be, a proficient practitioner who is able to employ empathy and emotional intelligence or a non-proficient practitioner.

Consider the therapist helping clients to do an exploration of their inner selves to heal – can you do this without understanding your client's heritage, beliefs, culture and life experiences?

Consider the teacher who ignores the cultural background and identity of the students they teach, so is unable to understand their lives or make sense of their behaviours.

The Iceberg Concept of culture by Edward T. Hall (1976), posits that a lot about culture is below the surface. There is surface, shallow and deep culture, visible and invisible. It is only by engaging with an individual's culture that we can understand and become well equipped as professionals.

The questions below are worth reflecting on at this stage.

Consider the reasons why you came into your field of work, particularly if it is a humanitarian field like healthcare, education or social work.

Was it to be loyal, and physically and psychologically available to a particular group of people more than others? To make a real difference in society to those who need it the most? Maybe you accidentally came into your field of practice while looking for a lucrative career with job prospects.

Maybe you chose the profession for other reasons and had not fully considered what the career entailed or what would be required of you.

Try writing down why you came into your profession, what values you hold and what you are hoping to achieve by reading this book. Do take the time to stop, really think and write with honesty.

Use the reflection notes at the end of this chapter to write down your answers. It will help you think about your beliefs, feelings and values and how you can take the initial steps to become culturally sensitive.

Only you can decide to be a culturally sensitive practitioner, and to do this you need to actively work towards it.

> Working effectively with diversity and becoming a culturally competent practitioner is a fundamental requirement for helping professionals. It is the key to becoming a robust and skilled worker at what you do.

Reflection notes

D: Decide to be a culturally sensitive practitioner.

Invite People to Talk about their Culture, Values, Beliefs and Experiences

To learn about a person or a group of people, you must be prepared to listen and hear. You must be willing and prepared to engage with them actively.

Curiosity is vital in professional practice. You need to be curious about others, their identities, their culture, the things they hold dear, and their lived experiences that have shaped them through life.

As professionals, we must not depend solely on a certain group of people's stories or experiences to understand or rationalize other people's behaviours. Everyone has their own stories, even within the same perceived culture groups. We need to move away from the 'one size fits all approach' or using 'one tape to measure all'.

At the risk of stating the obvious, carrying out any form of humanitarian work or interventions in people's lives, be it counselling or caring for the vulnerable, requires the act of 'individualizing'.

This is a common principle in the healthcare services all over the world, and individualizing means taking the time to learn about each person, their wishes and feelings and needs before tailoring your intervention to meet them in a person-centred manner.

Information is needed in whichever field of service you find yourself in – social care, healthcare, adult or children's services, education or public services.

You should allow service users, patients and clients to educate you on how to relate to and work with them. You can learn so much from service users by hearing their stories, which helps formulate interventions. Let service users tell you their individual stories.

The old saying 'knowledge is power' is very relevant to this letter of the acrostic poem.

Let me tell you the story of my life

Relying on X or Y to tell you the story of Z, or allowing the actions of one person or group to dictate the story of another is dangerous and unethical practice.

When we invite people or service users to speak to us about their experiences, it is crucial to listen to all perspectives, including individuals or communities who may be marginalized or overlooked, and to engage in an open and non-judgemental manner.

This allows us to listen to, hear and understand the stories of others and, when required, intervene more effectively in their lives.

As a professional, you should listen from a position of curiosity, acceptance and empathy to hear what is said to you and empathize. You listen not just for the fun of listening, but to seize the opportunity to acquire knowledge and skills about things which you may know little about, or may have misunderstood.

Through listening, you can also learn to challenge issues around cultural diversity constructively. Consider attending training on active listening and engagement to learn how to listen and hear, empathize, and respond in positive ways. As a social work student, I came across the motivational interviewing (MI) technique developed by Miller and Rollnick (2002) and fell in love with it due to its simplicity. The model was developed for interventions with service users affected by drug and alcohol misuse, and has since been adapted for use in child and family social work, among other things. It provides vital elements for successful interaction that influence positive change. The MI model is an approach that collaborates with the service user in making decisions about their behaviour change or future. It is a strengths-based approach which employs empathy, and utilizes active listening skills and affirmation among other strategies to create awareness and develop consistency with the clients.

The concept of 'reflective listening' is also helpful to consider here.

It is one of the essential skills required when you invite people to talk about themselves and their experiences. There is intrinsic value in being curious and learning about other cultures.

It enriches your knowledge and broadens your perspective. Your expertise becomes versatile.

Many make a huge mistake by classifying people of colour together – as black people, Asian people, Latinos and so on. Two people who share the same skin tone, appearance, hair and accent may have entirely different cultures, beliefs, values and life experiences. For example, the cultural attributes and worldviews of black people in the United States, the United Kingdom, the Caribbean Islands, and Africa vary widely regardless of having the same skin colour.

It is essential to learn about an individual's unique self. The best way is to *invite people to talk about their own cultures, values, beliefs, and experiences.*

When you talk, you are only repeating what you already know, but if you listen, you may learn something new. (Dalai Lama)

The reflection notes at the end of the chapter will help you to write down ways in which you can employ open-mindedness and curiosity in your day-to-day interactions and practice reflective listening. How do you think you can achieve this? Do you think you will need help from peers from different backgrounds?

Relying on X or Y to tell you the story of Z or the actions of a person/group to dictate the story of others is dangerous and unethical in any area of work, particularly in the humanitarian field of practice.

Reflection notes

I: Invite people to talk about their culture, values, beliefs and experiences.

Value Service Users' History, Individuality and Differences

I t is one thing to *acquire* information to enhance your knowledge, it's *using* this information that is the key to building cultural competence.

Helping professionals often have and maintain custody of service users' medical records and details about their lives which they manage on a day-to-day basis.

By sharing their history, stories and those things they hold dear – the experiences that have shaped them and continue to shape them – service users, patients and clients make themselves vulnerable to you.

As professionals working with these vulnerable clients, we need to value and respect this information, and the client's decision to volunteer it. The information and experiences they share may or may not be familiar to you, and may differ from your own experiences immensely.

Remember, *value* and *respect* are the key words here.

Take care not to minimize, reduce or undermine those values and experiences, or the differences you see.

You do not have to like or go along with the perspective you are presented with. You only need to acknowledge and try to understand it, and make sense of those experiences that have shaped the life of your patient or service user.

The essential skill required here for dedicated professionals is to remain curious and open-minded.

As a black social work professional, I have observed some white colleagues keeping interactions to a bare minimum or choosing not to interact with colleagues from black and ethnic minority groups.

I sometimes struggle to understand how such practitioners can carry out successful, robust interventions with vulnerable children and young people from different cultural backgrounds. I believe that helping professionals who dislike and hold back from interacting with people of different cultures and races will be seriously impeded from providing any meaningful intervention to vulnerable service users.

Undermining or ignoring people's cultures, beliefs and experiences diminishes them psychologically and can lower their self-esteem, impacting their emotional and mental health. I presume that this is not the aim of any dedicated professional.

In professions that seek to make positive change in society, there is a fundamental need to first connect with people, even in small ways. We should value the service user's history, individuality and difference.

Now use the reflection notes at the end of the chapter to detail practical steps you can take to show others that you value and appreciate them, and respect their culture.

> Undermining people's cultures, beliefs and experiences diminishes them psychologically and can lower their self-esteem, impacting their emotional and mental health.

Reflection notes

V: Value service users' history, individuality and differences.

Explore Clients' Realities and Show Curiosity

Having gathered as much information as you can about others, including your service users, you need to weigh up, reason and actively evaluate the information you have received.

Remember, this is your service user or patient's lived experience. For some, it will be a stark bitter reality. Some vulnerable people, including children and young people, will have experienced an awful lot in their lives. They may have lived through much more than you and other professionals who are aiming to support them. They may have experienced severe childhood trauma, abuse, neglect or loss of childhood. When thinking of the kinds of support some vulnerable children need, sometimes it is not primarily an *age* factor you need to consider but an *experience* factor. Once brought into care, children may further suffer the trauma of loss and separation from their loved ones and close family. Informed interventions can only be achieved from an in-depth exploration of the issues.

All individuals in society require sensitive interactions during encounters, both on a personal and a professional level, regardless of their culture, background and protected characteristics.

This can only be achieved through some degree of curiosity to understand and appreciate their individual stories. Everyone has their own life story, life experiences and challenges which they are grappling with.

When working with vulnerable children, networks of professionals including social workers, teachers, therapists, healthcare workers and foster carers must remember that, regardless of the abuse a child has experienced before coming into care, they still have a deep-rooted bond with their families. There could be emotions they may never share with the professionals working with them. Regardless of the dire circumstances that may have led children into the system, they naturally still love their families, mums, dads, siblings, in ways that professionals may never quantify.

This little detail is sometimes overlooked by those working with these children. The experiences of these vulnerable children may sometimes be unique, unfamiliar or just not understood by professionals of other cultures working with them. This is okay; we are all learners in a multicultural world.

A deeper exploration of the experiences of people from other cultures is very much needed when carrying out interventions with them. Vulnerable adults from diverse backgrounds, for example, may struggle with culture adaptations but lack the capacity to vocalize this or are too shy to speak out.

Helping professionals are often very busy, so it is always a challenge to deeply explore service users' cultures and experiences to create better connections. You should, however, attempt to do so wherever it's possible. In the early days of working with a patient or service user, your ability to show empathy can be put to the test – are you able to put yourself in the other person's shoes and feel their pain? Can you relate to those sad, deep and sometimes heart-wrenching life stories of your vulnerable service users from different cultural backgrounds? If so, how?

Empathy remains central to positive human interaction, particularly in the helping professions.

Dan Hughes, psychologist and founder of dyadic developmental psychotherapy, advocates a deep connection to service users' plights to create positive behaviour change. This means connecting to the experiences of service users through meaningful interactions in order to get a flavour of them, which in turn leads to meaningful change.

As helping professionals, we should show an active interest in people's lived experiences, cultures and beliefs, seek to understand their vulnerabilities and show a genuine desire to support them in overcoming their challenges. This is called having a caring attitude, being a considerate and thoughtful human being. Professions like social work, healthcare and teaching are caring professions.

Undertaking some early research into how best to support service users is vital, and should start with the service users themselves. For example, in children's services, professionals should refer to the child's voice, particularly children from black and other minority ethnic backgrounds whose voices often get lost. This advice may sound ordinary and mundane, but it is not.

One of the significant challenges facing children's services today is the loss of the voice of the children and young people in interventions that affect them. This is more so for children from minority ethnic or diverse backgrounds which professionals are not familiar with, or lack cultural knowledge of.

Sometimes these children's voices are lost, and with this their identities. It is only when we are knowledgeable about those things that mean much to the person we are supporting that we can achieve great success with our interventions.

In children's services and education, preserving children and young people's identity is key to building their self-esteem, which enables them to thrive and achieve despite everything they have gone through.

Specialists should strive to explore service users' realities, showing professional curiosity.

Using the reflection notes at the end of this chapter, detail some points that stood out for you.

Have you had instances where you have had to connect to a client's sad feelings or trauma or stories about them experiencing discrimination?

You can close your eyes at this point and think back; can you stand in their shoes for a short while? How does it feel to be the vulnerable person, or the person of difference, who is struggling to be heard and understood?

How will you support or empower your colleague or service user who experiences discrimination/racism?

Helping professionals need to be curious and carry out a robust exploration of their service users' experiences to make an impact. At this stage, the professional's ability to demonstrate empathy can be put to the test – are you able to put yourself in the other person's shoes and feel their pain?

Reflection notes

E: Explore clients' realities and show curiosity.

Reflect on the Information and Knowledge Received

The act of casting your mind back to question and evaluate your performance is often described as 'critical reflection'. Reflecting regularly on events and performances helps to broaden and enhance your communication skills as well as your professional skills to carry out interventions.

It contributes to your continuing professional development and increases your ability to analyse situations and make judgements around complex day-to-day work undertaken with service users (Schon 1983).

Critical reflection is a reasoning process, a conscious effort to think, to probe yourself and analyse events. Through critical reflection, you regularly question your interventions and your response to issues and circumstances. It enables you to explore your feelings and ways you can do things better next time. For example:

'What am I proud of today?'
'What can I do better next time?'
'What do I need to change in my way of working?'

In his book *Mindsight* (2010), Dan Siegel introduces interpersonal neurobiology – the study of the relationship between the mind, body and social interactions. He talks about the human reflective ability to perceive one's own mind as well as the minds of others, and to feel empathy for them. He describes the mind's power to change the physical brain's functioning, focusing on the internal world to modify 'diving into the sea within ourselves'. We essentially undergo a deep self-probing and reasoning process.

Critical reflection is essential for working with diversity because it can help you connect with your thought processes, including your emotional needs, to interact in a more socially acceptable manner, as a professional. It enables you to challenge yourself and your thinking to find new ways of working.

You can connect to those values, biases and prejudices, including those stories you were told growing up, relating to how they have shaped and continue to shape your perspective in your personal and professional life.

Reflection allows you to be self-aware and to remain balanced and objective in your professional interventions.

As helping professionals, we need to ensure that we do not let unfair judgements or preconceived notions be an influencing factor. We should not hesitate to challenge ourselves and others, even though this can be a painful exercise.

In their book on critical reflection, *Critical Thinking for Social Work*, Keith Brown and Lynne Rutter (2008) suggest that critical thinking can sometimes be challenging, threatening and anxiety-provoking, leading to unpleasant consequences or responses from other people.

As a practitioner, you should recognize your core feelings and seek help to address any events impacting negatively on your emotional wellbeing. You should use management, mentor or peer supervision to support yourself.

At the critical reflection stage, you can begin to form a new worldview after reflecting, processing and making sense of the information provided to you by service users. Try looking back at your performance, essentially debriefing yourself in order to make your practice and interventions better – consider aspects of your work that relate to anti-oppression and anti-discrimination.

When someone chooses to lay their lived experiences and feelings at your feet, there are usually deep feelings associated with this. They maybe in need of help, support, understanding or affirmation, and your role is to give that help and support.

The same applies within the education sector. When a student trusts their lecturer or college tutor with their learning, they expect a conducive and effective learning environment that is free of bias, judgement and discrimination. You cannot educate effectively if you are not understanding or communicating effectively with your students.

Social work authors Sue Thompson and Neil Thompson (2023) advocate the need for social work professionals to develop Schon's models of 'reflecting in action' (during) and 'reflecting on action' (after) so that the outcome of reflection benefits service users promptly during the intervention and not just retrospectively.

Doing so will involve the ability to reflect, think on your feet and act promptly, so where you become aware of issues relating to oppression and discrimination, you are able to act on them during your interaction.

In the autumn of 2020, a popular street dance troupe called Diversity gave a powerful performance on the TV show *Britain's Got Talent*. It aimed to summarize in dance form some of the key events affecting society in 2020.

Their performance reflected on the murder of George Floyd and the Black Lives Matter movement, as well as the Covid-19 pandemic – two of the main issues affecting society at the time. It would be impossible for history to ignore this. The UK's communications regulator Ofcom received more than 25,000 complaints from viewers about the performance, which dramatized the horrible murder. The rationale for the complaints was that *Britain's Got Talent* was not the 'right stage' for highlighting this. I agree with the leader of Diversity Ashley Banjo who responded to this accusation by saying:

> Why can we talk about a multitude of other issues yet me as a creative and an artist, with something that has affected me, impacted me deeply and also been global news for the past month, I'm not allowed to talk about it? (Heaf 2020)

I personally thought that the performance was a creative piece of dance art that highlighted racism and the Black Lives Matter (BLM) movement. The whole presentation was deeply reflective and should have been applauded. These complaints were dismissed, thank goodness for sanity!

The reflection notes at the end of the chapter will help you do some reflective exercises. Cast your mind back to an incident that happened to you in the past relating to discrimination or racism. Try to answer the following questions:

- What happened?
- What were your feelings or reaction to it?
- What was good and bad?
- What sense can you make of it?
- What have you learned?

'I feel proud that we [Diversity] have become a bit of a symbol for something that I want to live up to. I want to be able to speak up – and not just about racism.' [Ashley Banjo, Diversity] (Heaf 2020)

Reflection notes

R: Reflect on information and knowledge received.

Scrutinize Yourself – Personal SWOT Analysis

(Strengths, Weaknesses, Opportunities, Threats)

Scrutinizing yourself involves carrying out a deep, honest examination of yourself to understand your personality, capabilities, limitations and learning needs. It means acknowledging your perspective on life, your values and beliefs concerning diversity or cultural diversity and how they might affect your practice – examining stereotypes, prejudices, assumptions, your attitude, words and actions.

As professionals, we must probe our conscious and unconscious prejudices and biases.

It is important to note here that most biases are implicit – *so we may hold attitudes towards people or associate stereotypes with them without our conscious knowledge.* In this section, it is worth noting that every one of us – regardless of race, culture or background – will have prejudices and beliefs that we may inherit from family and peers or absorb from wider society.

Here is a short story that is very close to home.

My father's perspective (may his soul rest in peace): Once upon a time, my father was on my case to get married soon as I was perceived to be at the age of marriage. And why not? I had finished my university degree, and I had, in fact, concluded my Master's degree, so nothing was stopping me from getting married. It was the next logical step, especially from the typical African (Nigerian) family perspective. A promising young daughter, having concluded her university education, is expected to get married to a responsible young man from a decent family, have children and live happily ever after! At this stage, my conversations with my dad – usually over the phone due to living far apart, even a continent away – included subtle reminders to find a husband!

The conversations always carried silent undertones that simply said: 'Have you got news for me?' In other words, 'When will you be bringing home a suitor/fiancé to introduce to us?' I also had the pleasure of hearing about other mates of mine from our hometown who had recently got married straight after university!

As the months and years passed by, these subtle conversations became more desperate. I was the first daughter of six children, which was of considerable significance.

He was looking forward to having that proud Daddy moment, like most fathers. The message was clear; it is time to get married! So, you can imagine the excitement I felt when I met someone, and I looked forward to telling my dad that I would make him proud! I rang up and said, 'Dad, I am getting married!' He was undoubtedly very pleased and immediately proceeded to ask where my fiancé was from, a typical question asked by the average Nigerian parent. I stated that he was from Spain.

My dad responded: 'Oh great, he lives in Spain, but where is he from? What village is he from? Where are his parents from?' My dad, of course, presumed that my fiancé was no doubt going to be a Nigerian, so he wanted to know what village or town my fiancé was from. Nigeria has four major geographical regions, Northern, Southern, Eastern and Western.

I am from the Eastern part of the country. Parents would usually prefer their children to marry someone from the same geographical region for proximity purposes and cultural similarities. The thought process is that their children would remain as close as possible to home and the things familiar to them after marriage. In Nigeria, a person is from a settlement where their parents, grandparents, great grandparents came from going back generations.

They are not actually from where they were born, as it is in the western world, unless they were born in their family lineage location or settlement. This was precisely why my dad asked where my fiancé and his parents were from. I continued to answer that they were all from Spain and then dropped the 'shock'. 'He is white from Spain; both his parents are white and from Spain too!'

The penny dropped, and it took my dad a few minutes to digest that information. You could most certainly hear the loud inaudible silence down the telephone line. He immediately came back to me saying, 'Oh no, there is no need to rush; marriage is not what you rush into; you need to take your time...'

My dad's response was a fascinating one from someone who had been advocating strongly for me to get married! He was now taking a back step because I had presented someone out of the norm, someone who was not only from a different geographical region in Nigeria, but indeed from another world in my dad's eyes! 'Oyibo' (a white man).

My dad was now advocating for me to slow down. He felt that I had settled for a white man because I was under pressure and unable to secure myself a black Nigerian man. He then said that he did not think it was a good idea for me to marry a man who was not the same as me, who did not understand our culture and was most certainly going to draw me further away from my family. My dad was a well-read and educated man, a civil engineer who obtained his doctorate at the age of 67, although, sadly, he died two years after. He, however, fulfilled his lifelong academic ambition as a person who valued education. I feel that my dad, although quite literate, operated under the scope of his knowledge and his lack of familiarity with interracial marriage or 'white culture'.

I was sure that my dad meant no harm by his advice; he had not met my fiancé at this time. He was simply sticking to what he knew, his familiar territory. I would like to posit that his perspective was formed by his feeling of uncertainty, his lack of knowledge and his preconceived notions. As an individual, he needed more education in this unknown area.

I am pleased to say that he did open himself to learn and when he eventually met my husband, he embraced him and they got on very well. As a matter of fact, in my dad's typical upfront and blunt manner, he stated when they met that I was lucky to find myself such a handsome husband!

This story's learning is that we all hold some form of bias due to cultural differences, traditions, family stories told to us and preconceived notions – they may only surface when faced with a particular scenario or event. None of us can shy away from this. We first and foremost need to recognize them and be open to learning to have a good shot at changing those views and preconceived ideas.

Before coming into the humanitarian field of social work, I studied business administration and worked in business banking for a short while. In business, you often use a SWOT analysis to evaluate business 'temperature', and to plan and develop effective business strategies. Companies look at the four core areas: strengths, weaknesses, opportunities and threats. They compare the internal factors (strengths and weaknesses) against external factors (opportunities and threats) to strategically position themselves for growth and development.

The SWOT analysis has been adapted and applied to social work and other practice areas in recent times. The idea is that professionals can carry out a personal SWOT analysis of themselves and effectively do the same examination that organizations do.

This will enable you to understand your strengths and weaknesses, and the threats to your growth and development, including opportunities available to you.

As a professional, you can consider your perspective, values, beliefs and understanding of diversity, and how they might affect your practice. As mentioned earlier, we need to think about the stories and values handed to us by our parents, grandparents and family lineage. Those stories we were told in our childhood that have stayed with us over time. We must consider how they have shaped us and continue to shape our lives. Everyone has something – as individuals, we all hold some form of bias.

Dr Robin DiAngelo, Professor of Education at the University of California and an expert in anti-racism and anti-bias, advocates for a deep understanding of self in tackling bias. She is the author of the bestselling book *White Fragility: Why it's So Hard for White People to Talk About Racism* (2018). Dr DiAngelo posits that white people are essentially born and bred into a system of inequality through no making of their own. It's an inculcated and internalized notion of superiority that white people just have – a fundamental white privilege that sprang from white supremacy. This is something that white people must acknowledge to help them understand racism.

Di Angelo further posits that anti-black bias is profoundly ingrained in the white culture – the notion that black people are inferior. The idea of inferiority is needed to maintain superiority, leading to racism (whether conscious or unconscious). The average four-year-old child soon learns that it is better to be white than black...that the system we live in portrays no inherent value in the perspectives and experiences of people of colour. According to DiAngelo, white people are not often taught about the feelings of loss associated with segregation and, subsequently, some can move from 'cradle to grave in racial segregation'.

Some white people choose to live in racial segregation, not interacting much or socializing with black people due to not seeing any value in doing so. And those closest to them, as well as society, have not shown or taught them the value in doing so.

DiAngelo surmises that people of colour's distrust in schools and institutions is rational, including black people's default view of white people as racists. This is due to decades of slavery, negative racial experiences and a long history of distrust. Unfortunately, this default view paints all white people with the same brush, and doesn't reflect reality.

She also refers to society's default to the reproduction of racism as a system failure which has continued for many generations.

As a social work professional, I find Dr DiAngelo's arguments very insightful and fascinating. They provide me with awareness of the fragility of white colleagues. They allude to the fact that one can become accustomed to privilege such that it can be extremely difficult to give it up; that it can feel highly repressive to be asked to share it. It certainly helped me to form a different perspective on the age-old problem of racism.

It is only in understanding the root of our prejudices that we can address problematic beliefs. It means that for us as professionals to reflect a truthful narrative of ourselves, we need to consider our psychosocial development and identify any learned behaviour that needs to change – and give some thought to how to create that change.

For example, by scrutinizing yourself, you may identify a strength in your ability to learn; you may identify a weakness in your knowledge and understanding of cultures beyond your own. By assessing your learning needs and pursuing training opportunities, you can address your weaknesses.

Following the worldwide protests over George Floyd's death and the turbulent racial climate in 2020, suggestions were made for British MPs to undertake mandatory training on unconscious bias. The suggestion was immediately met with resistance by several Conservative MPs (BBC News online 2020). The opposition was criticised by Labour MP Diane Abbott, who tweeted in August 2020: 'Nothing says bias like someone who absolutely refuses to discuss the possibility that they might be biased.'

If we think back to the SWOT, there were clear opportunities for learning and growth among public servants accountable to a society of diverse people.

As a professional, you should be able to challenge deeply entrenched prejudices, stereotypes and generational 'hand-me-downs' from your family. Consider how they have shaped and continue to shape your perspective in your personal and professional life.

'Truly engaging with diversity and inclusion feels personal, disruptive, and emotional' (Ross & Hills 2020). Acknowledging white privilege, the possibility of conscious or unconscious bias, is fundamental in engaging with diversity and promoting justice and equality.

> Racism hurts people of colour 24/7; interrupting it is more important than my feelings, ego, or self–image. (DiAngelo 2018)

Regardless of race and culture, every individual has their individual beliefs, prejudices and biases that they are either born into or are passed down from family generations, or otherwise handed by society at large.

Reflection notes

S: Scrutinize yourself – personal SWOT analysis.
Write down your thoughts under the four SWOT headings:

Your strengths as an individual or a professional around working with diversity.

....

....

....

Your areas of weaknesses.

....

....

....

The opportunities immediately available to you to mitigate your perceived weaknesses.

....

....

....

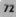

The perceived threats around you.

....

....

....

Identify Strategies to Aid Your Work

n this chapter, you should ask yourself the following questions:

- How do I, as a professional, rewrite history and change my racial construct to embrace diversity?
- As a helping professional, how do I engage with authenticity and reality?
- How can I develop an empathic disposition towards people of difference, disadvantaged people, and the less privileged?
- How do I ensure that my personal views assimilated over time do not obstruct my work with clients who are different from me?
- How do I acknowledge, respect and engage with diversity?

Healthcare and social care professionals have a duty to

promote anti-discriminatory and anti-oppressive practice; it is one of the core principles in this field and hence a non-negotiable area.

Professionals must identify and access training, research, management and mentor supervision and apply these aspects in practice. I imagine that a fundamental requirement of any profession is to constantly engage in continued professional development to improve practice. In social work, professionals can use available models of practice in supporting vulnerable children and families, and adults from diverse backgrounds. They can also use models such as the Signs of Safety (SOS) to look at what is working well in practice, particularly in interacting and solving problems for children and families from different backgrounds. One of the parenting and caregiving attachment models called the Secure Base which is used by some local authorities in the UK provides a straightforward approach for considering and meeting the needs of vulnerable children. Dimension 3 of the Secure Base model (Acceptance – Building the child's self-esteem) and dimension 4 (Co-operation – Helping the child feel effective) can help promote anti-oppressive and anti-discriminatory caregiving for vulnerable, looked-after children.

The Social Graces illustrative tool developed by John Burnham, Alison Roper-Hall and colleagues (2012) to address social inequality presented an extended version of the Equality Act 2010 protected characteristics. It is a helpful reminder of those diverse characteristics that form an individual's identity, although they may not necessarily be exhaustive, especially with new emerging orientations. A BASW article by Rebekah Pierre in July 2020 is also a good reminder of the Social Graces model. The idea of naming the power differentials helps professionals identify and address their biases and preconceptions. Most professionals will have areas within the Equality Act protected characteristics and Social Graces which pose a challenge and impact their ability to work in a culturally competent manner. Practitioners should research and explore widely to identify strategies that can aid them in this area of work. Helping professionals must develop and nurture a learning attitude. The famous saying 'life is a learning curve' remains very relevant. Continued learning is required to ensure that service users' best interests are at the forefront of our practice.

Practical strategies could be liaising with and obtaining information and support from your colleagues from other backgrounds to inform your work. This will mitigate situations where professionals are worried about how to approach issues or getting things wrong.

It is often the norm to underestimate black colleagues' education, knowledge and skills, particularly when they did not study in the big nations in the western world, such as the UK, US and Canada. Regardless of where they are from, be they black or white, each individual or professional has unique talents that should be given a fair opportunity to soar. We are surrounded by a rich diversity of people, skills, talents and abilities. Not taking good advantage of, enjoying and appreciating the benefits of these is a shame. Equality in the workplace is about promoting all professionals, regardless of their cultural background, to grow progressively alongside each other. Most workplaces lack anti-racism policies or strategies that actively promote equality and diversity. Organizations should be deliberate and show active interest and commitment to tackling inequality and racism. They can ask for help and support from the black and ethnic minority group of staff within their establishment. There is available evidence that when staff feel valued, respected, and supported in their work environment by their leaders, there is a huge probability of higher productivity and innovation (West & Richter 2007).

The equality legislation in most countries provides a direction of travel for anti-discriminatory practice; however, the desired outcomes can only be achieved when leaders intentionally create and implement suitable strategies. There have been calls for racism to be tackled or treated separately from the other protected characteristics. The notion is that even though there is no hierarchy in inequality, combating racism should be prioritized due to the deeply rooted nature of it spanning over decades. There is some merit in this but it may not be easy to achieve in our society as it is today.

Useful strategies could include liaising with and obtaining information and support from your colleagues or clients from diverse backgrounds.

Reflection notes

I: Identify strategies to aid your work.

Train Yourself to Treat People, Children and Families Individually

Having gone through all the steps set out above, you can now begin to put the identified strategies in place and employ your acquired skills and knowledge in practice. This means developing the act of treating individuals, fellow professionals, families and service users from other cultural backgrounds, individually not collectively. This is where professionals depart from the approach of using; 'one measuring tape to measure all' and instead step into individualized one-to-one interventions with service users. This prevents humanitarian workers like social workers, teachers and perhaps other professionals from falling into the trap of generalizing or succumbing to common statements such as:

'X Y Z children are usually feral.'

'X Y Z children are aggressive and violent.'

'Black children don't fit in here.'

'Black children need to be placed with black carers.'

'Unaccompanied asylum seekers are dangerous.'

'Immigrants or foreigners come into our country and take our jobs.'

Statements like these are uninformed and do little to enhance the plight of vulnerable children, young, people and adults. Instead, they stigmatize the already disadvantaged groups before they've even had a chance to speak up or defend themselves.

Working with diversity and becoming a culturally sensitive practitioner means that a professional is in tune with the fact that the vulnerable service users they work with may come from different backgrounds, diverse situations and circumstances, and they all need equal help and support.

Every person has their own personality, history, culture and worldview that have shaped them over time into the person they have become today. For example, when working with vulnerable children, particularly looked-after children, we can see how their home life or general life experience has shaped them before coming into the care system. This can manifest in the form of trauma-led behaviours observed by the professionals working with them. It is essential to remind ourselves that those children were not necessarily born that way. It is important to note that with a lot of warmth and nurture from their carers, they can thrive again. This means that professionals still have that window of opportunity to make a significant positive difference that can go a long way to influence these children's future direction. Children from all backgrounds can be supported to break out of negative behaviour patterns and pursue the route to enjoying and achieving. It is only when professionals connect deeply with individual circumstances that they can carry out robust interventions that create change.

> You must connect in order to correct. (Dan Hughes in a lecture on dyadic developmental psychotherapy)

Professionals must seek a clear and reasonable understanding of their service users' culture and circumstances to be able to tailor their work to meet those needs. Social workers, particularly in children's services, should train themselves to explore vulnerable children and young people's identities and cultures. This enables them to put together a detailed life story from the very onset of their work and, most importantly, share these valuable insights with fellow professionals and carers. A well-compiled life story essentially helps professionals to work well together to support children's identity, which is fundamental in realizing positive outcomes for vulnerable children. All professionals need to be proactive in identifying relevant and available resources on anti-racism and cultural competence. A Community Care article by Tina

Amongi (2020), 'Food is a marker of identity: Supporting foster children's cultural heritage', highlights how social workers and foster carers should pay serious attention to children's cultural identity to avoid 'cultural dislocation'. There is a considerable emphasis on the social worker's critical role in ensuring that looked-after children maintain their identity and remain in touch with their heritage.

Social workers should strive to obtain and collate adequate information on the identities of looked-after children which they can share with the prospective carers to ensure that their cultural needs are adequately met. Social workers remain accountable, so it is important to display the appropriate skills required to safeguard vulnerable children and adults, including promoting their cultures. This means that social workers must recognize the multi-dimensional layers of diversity, including the protected characteristics such as race, disability, class, economic status, age, gender, faith and so on. They should bear in mind that one person's life experience may include oppression and marginalization while another person's experience may be of privilege and power. This is what shapes a person's identity and general outlook on life. It is indeed a mandatory requirement for social workers to be proficient in cultural competence, developing the ability to treat people from all backgrounds individually, fairly and equitably. They learn to balance power to impact service users positively in real time. The same applies to professionals in healthcare who also deal with vulnerable people, both adults and children of all ages, all of whom require to be treated fairly, equally and with dignity. Education professionals are also key in this discourse because they are responsible for training the future generation. Children need to understand not just the functional but the dysfunctional workings of society, including how they can adjust to and manage their lives within it.

Professionals, particularly those working with vulnerable looked after children and young people, should train themselves to explore their service users' identity and culture to put together a detailed and accurate life story.

Having done all there is to stand, as a proficient professional you must stand firm and be a culturally competent practitioner.

Reflection notes

T: Train yourself to treat people, children and families individually.

Yield to Culturally Sensitive Practice

This is the final domain of the Diversity Acrostic Poem. It simply means that as a progressive professional or a humanitarian worker wishing to be robust and competent in practice, you must yield to culturally sensitive practice. It is the baseline for professionals dealing with humans. In the profession of social work, for example, you cannot claim to put a child in the centre and work in their best interest if you consciously or unconsciously ignore or minimize their culture or the culture of those like them. Your practice could effectively be described as superficial and just scraping the surface. Having finally navigated the Diversity Acrostic Poem – the individual letters, and the associated phrases – you must form a view on cultural diversity and choose to interact and work positively with this.

Having done all there is to stand, you must stand firm and become a culturally competent practitioner. You must understand culture as dynamic, you must challenge stereotypes and reject prescribed cultural understanding in favour of focusing on individual circumstances to provide positive interventions. You must own your practice and train others. In so doing, you become a professional leader in your field of practice.

> Lack of knowledge or understanding of a particular client's culture, family dynamics, or worldview often gives rise to resistance and could delay or harm the social work intervention process. (Comas-Díaz & Jacobson 1991)

Professionals must seek to recognize and have a reasonable understanding of the worldviews of their colleagues, clients and service users to interpret presented behaviours and proffer enduring solutions.

Every child matters. Every person matters. All lives matter. Let Black Lives Matter too.

Diversity is the norm in nature. Being part of a minority is being part of the whole.

Reflection notes

Y: Yield to culturally sensitive practice.

HOW CAN BLACK PEOPLE COLLABORATE IN PROMOTING ANTI-RACIST PRACTICE?

I t is often very costly for black people to challenge racism; hence they need their white colleagues to support them. As a black person, you recognize at a very early age that you are not part of the predominant culture, you are outside the norm, you are always seen as 'the other' because of the colour of your skin.

Challenging racism in the workplace can frequently label black people as 'troublesome', 'difficult', 'the victim', and so on. It can also lead to stigmatization, stagnancy in the workplace and job loss. Regardless, black people must continue to raise awareness and challenge racism when it occurs because not doing so contributes to racial discrimination.

Some black people choose not to speak about racism because they are under the misapprehension that discrimination will not be directed at them. This group feel that they are somewhat 'special' or 'superior' to other black people or people subjected to racism. The notion is that they are more accepted for whatever reasons. Some of these reasons could be because they see themselves as having lighter skin colour, being of mixed-race background or being born and educated in the western world, or they have a white American or British accent. The list goes on... Black people should show a unified front towards a common goal and avoid division.

Some black professionals separate themselves from fellow black colleagues to fit into the white majority group. This could be to situate themselves in their quest for belonging, to access better work roles or ascend to higher job positions, among other reasons. I believe that racism thrives because black people do not come together with one voice and stand firmly against it. Black people are not as unified as they could be. This little detail is not missed in society, and it remains a recipe for continued racial discrimination. In the workplace, we can be seen competing against each other to prove ourselves and secure our positions.

Some black people are under the illusion or false security that they fit in better, while others feel that they are liked better, are more established, and hence untouchable. Black people and other minority ethnic groups need to unite and look out for each other because we are unquestionably the less privileged in society. That is the stark reality. The divide between black people is apparent in workplaces, where black people are sometimes used to invalidate discrimination or racism reports. For example, when a victim reports racism, the perpetrator is soon observed to be attempting to work better with the next black person within the team to portray themselves to the contrary. Consequently, when that black person is called on to speak about their own experiences with such a perpetrator, they will immediately give guarded, glowing feedback simply to safeguard their job or position. Perpetrators can then walk free of any consequences and continue to repeat the same behaviour, knowing that they will suffer no meaningful repercussions. Such a scenario enables racism to thrive.

Another group of black people choose to disassociate themselves from race issues to avoid the associated emotional implications. This group prefer to focus on their jobs, career growth and so on, which is understandable. However, it is essential to create some space to educate white people non-judgementally about racism, without giving up too quickly.

Black leaders and managers should not take the 'climbing ladder' down once they have reached a leadership position. They should mentor and support other black staff up the ladder and do so bravely and unapologetically. This is because they are all in the same disadvantaged group. Leaders should intentionally support skilled and well-deserving black colleagues to achieve their full potential and fill positions of management and leadership. This will enable these staff to contribute to influencing positive change too. A leader or a manager's key role is to recognize skills and talents and ensure they are nurtured to their full potential. Talent is not limited to a specific group. Once you recognize skills and talent, flag them up and get others to join you to promote the same so that high workplace productivity is achieved. An environment of increased productivity is achieved through inclusion, supportiveness and safety.

Black people must unite against a common goal and speak out in one voice against injustices to them and their colleagues in minority groups. They should strive to challenge racism constructively, knowing what battles to fight today and what struggles to leave for another day.

Within this discourse, bravery is required and diplomacy is needed. Standing up with integrity for what is right is an excellent place to start. We should be bold in standing up for each other to achieve justice and fair play in the world.

A LETTER
TO READERS

Dear Readers,

I hope this letter finds you well.

I wanted to commiserate with you all concerning the tragic
murder of George Floyd in the US in May 2020. This act, seen
as an act of racism around the world, was a sore wound and
heartbreaking for humanity. The incident affected us all whether
we are of the black, brown or white background. I could not watch
the full eight-minute and forty-six-second video of the murder
because of its distressing and deeply saddening nature.

This murder is not an isolated incident because there were many
before him and indeed more after him. These incidents have
been ongoing for decades, not just in the US and the UK but in
other countries — covert and overt racism, systematic limitations,
restrictions and killings.

My fellow black social work, healthcare, education and other professionals, hating racists is not the solution. It is about challenging racism constructively while providing education where required and as many times as needed.

My question to you is: How are you challenging racism? Are you challenging it constructively? Do you strive to educate on anti-racism? Are you facilitating and supporting positive change?

My fellow white social work, healthcare, education and other professionals, black people need the empathy of white people, their support and understanding around the issue of racism so that black lives can begin to matter too.

My question to you is: Are you consciously aware of your privileges? How are you embracing diversity and promoting inclusion? Are you facilitating and supporting positive change? Or are you obstructing change?

SUMMARY

The benefits of diversity, the importance of preserving a person's identity and the need for cultural competence in our society cannot be over-emphasized. Valuing and promoting diversity is an important aspect of making equality a reality. As individuals, we cannot deny the prevalence of white privilege in society. The murder of George Floyd accentuated and brought some light to supposedly dark-shaded areas and created more engagement with the Black Lives Matter movement, and rightly so. There is a huge responsibility for organizations and leaders to lead the way in this field of discourse by setting out visions, work policies and action plans that enable diversity to thrive. As Gloria Tabi says, 'A truly diverse and inclusive workplace will fundamentally challenge rigid processes that don't serve the marginalised' (Tabi 2021).

Education, healthcare staff, social workers, foster carers,

public servants, politicians and so on must all pay closer attention to the diversity around them. They should not be anxious or too apprehensive to discuss sensitive subjects like racism, or conscious, unconscious bias. Ignorance is no longer an excuse.

As mentioned earlier in this book, in late 2020 in the UK, the media reported a prominent public member, the FA Chairman, being forced to resign due to inappropriate language around diversity. Public servants, social care, social work professionals and the public need to reframe their language. Language use must be purposeful and respect how individuals, groups and communities choose to be identified.

In humanitarian professions such as social work and education, a lack of knowledge, understanding and respect for service users' culture and beliefs is detrimental to the professions' ethos and could become costly. Social workers, for example, need to engage positively with diversity, and their voices should be heard audibly advocating for anti-racism and equality. Social work is a profession that is fundamentally rooted in anti-oppressive and anti-discriminatory practices. Racism is a huge societal problem, and a lack of criticism can be deemed as complicity.

In early 2021, the Duke and Duchess of Sussex in England, Prince Harry and Meghan, granted an interview with US talk show host Oprah Winfrey. The interview, which was watched by millions in the UK, US and around the world, alluded to

Meghan, the first mixed-race member of the royal family in the UK, experiencing racism. The discussions showed that racial discrimination poses a clear and present danger in society. It showed the impact that racism or the perception of racism can have on a person's emotional and mental wellbeing.

According to Meghan's admission, her mental health had deteriorated quite significantly, which is not an unfamiliar ground because racism harms people of colour deeply.
It needs to be challenged and addressed right from the top, across institutional and leadership pipelines. Anti-racism education is critically required at all levels to support working positively with diversity. There needs to be a radical evolution to change the future narrative.

Following his inauguration as the 46th President of the United States of America, Joe Biden outlined his focus for the first one hundred days in office, which included plans to address racial inequality in the country. He stated: 'This is the time to address systemic racism and inequity.' Although this is coming decades too late, it may seem like a new dawn in the country and may hold some glimmer of hope. Biden aptly described the murder of George Floyd as 'a knee on the neck of justice'. He further stated that addressing racial inequality was not a one-department mission but a whole government department approach.

Indeed, it is safe to say that tackling inequality, systemic, or everyday racism in our society at large and our world today remains a whole community job. The struggle should not be only for those affected. Racism is a societal problem.

According to Biden, 'We are all God's Children; we should treat others as we like to be treated ourselves. All people are created equal and have a right to be treated equally' (Maule 2021). I agree, we are all indeed God's children...

'Systemic racism is corrosive, destructive and costly.'
He further stated that it is time to let go of notions such as: 'If you succeed, I fail. If you get ahead, I fall behind. If you get the job, I lose mine. And maybe worse of all, if I hold you down, I lift myself up.'

He concluded: 'When we lift each other up, we are all lifted up.'

Joe Biden effectively advocated for unity among diverse people and the embracing of diversity and inclusion in Society. His argument sums up this book.

In addition, Amanda Gorman, Inaugural Poet at the US President's Inauguration in January 2021 said: 'We are striving to forge our union with purpose. To compose a country committed to all cultures, colours, characters, and conditions of man.'

I hope that I have used the Diversity Acrostic Poem to convey a meaningful message around diversity and cultural competence. Professionals around the world must begin

to rewrite history to engage in positive communication,
collaboration and grounded interventions. We are living in
a revolving world with very unprecedented and spectacular
unknowns and there is limited time to make a positive impact.

Thank God for making this book a reality.

PROFESSIONALS' FEEDBACK

'The Diversity Acrostic Poem creatively acronymises the word diversity and effectively draws out some of the key principles of cultural sensitivity.' (Wayne Reid, Professional Officer, British Association of Social Workers)

'The Diversity Acrostic Poem is a creative way of finding the simplicity in the complexity of diversity. It will be a useful tool to encourage cultural awareness.' (Siobhan Maclean, social work publisher, Kirwin Maclean)

'The Diversity Acrostic Poem book is not only timely and innovative, it is also refreshingly inspiring, bold and challenges. Thank you for writing this book. I look forward to having it and would encourage everyone to read it.' (Ellen Holroyd, social work practitioner, Surrey)

'The book is written with passion, the Diversity Acrostic

Poem is a great working tool, and there are some real gems of wisdom.' (Jill Seeney, children's book author and Fostering Development Manager, West Sussex County Council)

'This book is an insightful and inspiring read that reflects on racism and diversity in a humane and creative way. The Diversity Acrostic Poem gives social work practitioners a helpful tool to use in tackling the inequalities many of the people we work with face every day in our unequal society.' (Adrian Rutledge, Social Work Practice Manager, West Sussex County Council)

'The Diversity Acrostic poem is an example of creative anti-racist social work practice. Racism and white privilege are perpetuated through division, paralysis and avoidance. Vivian's work challenges us not to turn away but to rise up and engage, with ourselves, with each other and with children and their families. Her work manages to be simple, inclusive and playful – it is an invitation to social work to be curious and creative. In her performance of the poem at a CoramBAAF practice forum, Vivian skillfully mobilized her insight, vulnerability and energy. It felt like a gift to us. I am sure social work colleagues will appreciate her work and her challenge.' (Louise Sims, Kinship Care and Fostering Consultant, CoramBAAF)

'Vivian's work on the issue of diversity and anti-racist social work is inspiring and timely...so many parallels with what is going on across the world and such a powerful tool to use.' (Yewukai Tsanga, Group Manager, Children Looked After)

'This book presents one of the most helpful explanations on diversity. It is filled with examples and strategies to assist social work professionals and clinicians. It is highly recommended.' (Elaine Williams, independent senior social work practitioner)

'The Diversity Acrostic Poem book is a creative and interesting approach to addressing the issue of diversity, inclusion and racism. The presentation and writing style are easy to read. The book aims to challenge social work practitioners, policymakers and the readers in general about the issue of social graces and the importance of diversity, equity and inclusion as a means of creating equal opportunities for practitioners and the children and families that we work with in social care. It showcases a creative way of entering a dialogue about ensuring that people from diverse backgrounds are offered the opportunity to share their ideas and perspectives and feel respected and appreciated.' (Toyin Sokale, Practice Manager, Children Looked After)

ABOUT THE AUTHOR

Vivian Okeze-Tirado is the Equality, Diversity and Inclusion Lead for West Sussex County Council Children Services. Prior to this, she was an Advanced Social Worker in the Fostering team for over seven years. She sat as a social work member of the Adoption Panel for two years. Vivian is a practice educator and facilitates social work training for social work practitioners and foster carers on the Secure Base model, diversity, cultural competence and Black Lives Matter, as well as other areas. Vivian's first degree was in linguistics, followed by a Master's degree in Business Administration – Management. Having sufficiently explored her initial career, Vivian decided to move into social work to pursue a more humanitarian career around improving the outcomes for vulnerable children and families. Vivian obtained her second Master's degree in Social Work from Brighton University in 2014. She is keen on social work research and practice development. She has developed useful materials for social workers and foster carers to enhance the experiences of children from all backgrounds. Vivian is the author of the Diversity Acrostic Poem and book. The poem is also published in the British Association of Social Workers book, *Outlanders: Hidden Narratives from Social Workers of Colour – An Anthology*. As a social worker of African origin, a wife and a mum, Vivian understands the importance of cultural competence in social work and other professions. She advocates strongly for justice, equality and inclusion.

PRACTICAL HELP AND SUPPORT FOR THE LESS PRIVILEGED

https://berrywell.org.uk

https://blacklivesmatter.com

https://redefineshop.co.uk

www.actionforchildren.org.uk

www.childline.org.uk

www.nspcc.org.uk

www.unicef.org.uk

FURTHER RESOURCES

Books

Alko, S. (2015). *The Case for Loving: The Fight for Interracial Marriage.* New York, NY: Arthur A. Levine Books.

Brooks, F. (2018). *All about Families.* London: Usborne Publishing.

Byers, G. (2020). *I Am Enough.* New York, NY: HarperCollins.

Eddo-Lodge, R. (2018). *Why I'm No Longer Talking to White People About Race.* London: Bloomsbury Publishing.

Guyton Hunt, I. (2020). *Black Culture Traditions – Visible and Invisible.* San Diego, CA: Cognella.

Hakim, A. (2019). *Black British History. New Perspectives.* London: Zed Books Illustrated.

Harrison, V. (2017). *Little Leaders. Bold Women in Black History.* London: Penguin Random House.

Holton, L. (1997). *A History of African American People.* Detroit, MI: Wayne State University Press.

Johnson, L. (2020). *You Should See Me in a Crown.* London: Scholastic Corporation.

Katz, K. (2002). *The Colors of Us*. New York, NY: Square Fish.

Lester, J. (2020). *Let's Talk About Race*. New York, NY: HarperCollins.

Lewis, D. & Awolaja, F. (2014). Black Children in Care: Health, Hair & Skin. Positive Image project.

Lindsay, B. (2019). *We Need to Talk About Race. Understanding the Black Experience in White Majority Churches*. London: Society for Promoting Christian Knowledge.

Love, J. (2018). *Julian is a Mermaid*. London: Walker Books.

Memory, J. (2019). *A Kid's Book About Racism*. Portland, OR: Kids Book About.

Moon, J.A. (2004). *A Handbook of Reflective and Experiential Learning: Theory and Practice*. London: Routledge Falmer.

Oluo, I. (2018). *So, You Want to Talk About Race*. New York, NY: Basic Books.

Reid, W. & Maclean, S. (2021). *Outlanders: Hidden Narratives from Social Workers of Colour*. Lichfield, Staffordshire: Kirwin Maclean Associates.

Saad, L. & DiAngelo, R. (2020). *Me and White Supremacy: How to Recognise Your Privilege, Combat Racism, and Change the World*. London: Quercus.

Siegel, D. (2010). *The Mindful Therapist: A Clinician's Guide to Mindsight and Neural Integration*. New York: W. W. Norton & Company.

Sissay, L. (2019). *My Name is Why*. Edinburgh: Canongate Books.

Thompson, N. (2006). *Anti-Discriminatory Practice*. London: Palgrave Macmillan.

Thompson, N. (2009). *Practicing Social Work. Meeting the Professional Challenge*. London: Palgrave Macmillan.

Thompson, N. (2011). *Promoting Equality: Working with Diversity and Difference* (third edition). London: Palgrave Macmillan.

Torrey, M. (2020). *What Lane?* New York, NY: Penguin Random House.

Useful websites

www.education-ni.gov.uk

www.equalityhumanrights.com/en/equality-act

www.gov.uk/government/organisations/department-for-education

www.legislation.gov.uk/ukpga/2010/15/section/4

https://onlinesocialwork.vcu.edu/blog/cultural-competence-in-social-work

www.researchinpractice.org.uk/children/publications/2017/july/confident-practice-with-cultural-diversity-frontline-briefing-2017

www.skillsforcare.org.uk/Leadership-management/developing-leaders-and-managers/Supporting-the-diverse-workforce-within-adult-social-care.aspx#WebinarSeries

www.socialworkengland.org.uk

www.youtube.com/watch?v=h7mzj0cVL0Q Deconstructing White Privilege with Dr Di Angelo

https://vottraining.co.uk

REFERENCES

Aljazeera News (2021). How many people have been killed by US police since George Floyd? www.aljazeera.com/news/2021/5/25/how-many-people-have-police-killed-since-george-floyd

Amongi, T. (2020). Food is a marker of identity: Supporting foster children's cultural heritage. Community Care. www.communitycare.co.uk/2020/10/30/food-marker-identity-supporting-foster-childrens-cultural-heritage

Ardern, J. (2018). Guardian News on YouTube. Contrasting styles: Trump and Ardern speak at UN. www.youtube.com/watch?v=iaHBuzZoYKQ

Ardern, J. (2019). CNN on Twitter. https://twitter.com/cnn/status/1108662634243678208

BBC News online (2020). Parliament: Tory MPs refuse unconscious bias training. www.bbc.co.uk/news/uk-politics-54282685

Boyne, J. (2006). *The Boy in the Striped Pyjamas*. London: Vintage Children's Classics.

British Association of Social Workers (2018). Professional Capabilities Framework for Social Work in England. www.basw.co.uk/system/files/resources/PCF%20Final%20Documents%20Overview%2011%20June%202018.pdf

Brown, K. & Rutter, L. (2008). *Critical Thinking for Social Work*. Exeter: Learning Matters.

Burnham, J. (2012). Developments in Social GRRRAAACCEEESSS: Visible–Invisible and Voiced–Unvoiced. In I.-B. Krause (ed.), *Culture and Reflexivity in Systemic Psychotherapy: Mutual Perspectives* (pp.139–160). London: Karnac.

Comas-Díaz, L. & Jacobsen, F.M. (1991). Ethnocultural transference and countertransference in the therapeutic dyad. *American Journal of Orthopsychiatry*, 61(3): 392–402. doi: 10.1037/h0079267.

DiAngelo, R. (2018). *White Fragility: Why it's So Hard for White People to Talk About Racism*. London: Allen Lane.

The Guardian (2022). The shameful strip search of Child Q. www.theguardian.com/news/audio/2022/mar/25/shameful-strip-search-of-child-q-today-in-focus-podcast

Hall, E. (1976). *Beyond Culture*. Garden City, NY: Anchor Press.

Heaf, J. (2020). Ashley Banjo: 'Britain isn't racist. But racism here is real.' *GQ Magazine*. www.gq-magazine.co.uk/gq-hype/article/ashley-banjo-diversity-interview

Helmore, E. & Smith, D (2022). Joe Biden says 'white supremacy is a poison' after Buffalo shooting. *The Guardian*, 17 May. www.theguardian.com/us-news/2022/may/17/joe-biden-buffalo-shooting-white-supremacist-lies

Kallehauge, K. (March 2021). How education sustains racial inequality and white supremacy. IMPAKTER. https://impakter.com/how-education-sustains-racial-inequality-and-white-supremacy

Maule, J. (2021). 'We're all God's children': President Biden signs executive order on racial equality. Christian News. https://premierchristian.news/en/news/article/we-re-all-god-s-children-president-biden-signs-executive-order-on-racial-equality

McGregor-Smith, R. (2017). Race in the workplace: The McGregor-Smith Review. Department for Business, Energy & Industrial Strategy.

Miller, W. & Rollnick, S. (2002). *Motivational Interviewing: Preparing People for Change* (second edition). New York, NY: Guilford Press.

Pierre, R. (2020). Social Graces: A practical tool to address inequality. www.basw.co.uk/media/news/2020/jul/social-graces-practical-tool-address-inequality

Ross, S. & Hills, S. (2020). Passion with no end: Where next for our diversity and inclusion work? The Kings Fund blog. www.kingsfund.org.uk/blog/2020/09/passion-no-end-where-next-our-diversity-and-inclusion-work

Schon, D. (1983). *The Reflective Practitioner. How professionals think in action.* London: Temple Smith.

Siegel, D. (2010). *Mindsight: The New Science of Personal Transformation.* New York, NY: Bantam.

Social Work England Professional Standards. www.socialworkengland.org.uk/standards/professional-standards

Tabi, G. (2021). Are Black and marginalised employees supported by diversity and inclusion policies? https://www.linkedin.com/pulse/black-marginalised-employees-supported-diversity-

Thompson, S. and Thompson, N. (2023). *The Critically Reflective Practitioner, 3rd edn.* London: Bloomsbury.

Ugwuegbula, L. (2020). The role of education in perpetuating racism and white supremacy: Rethinking the Eurocentric Curriculum. Manitoba Canada: Samuel Centre of Social Connectedness. www.socialconnectedness.org/the-role-of-education-in-perpetuating-racism-and-white-supremacy-rethinking-the-eurocentric-curriculum

Virginia Commonwealth University (2019). Why cultural competence in social work is a vital skill. https://onlinesocialwork.vcu.edu/blog/cultural-competence-in-social-work

West, M.A. & Richter, A.W. (2007). Climates and Cultures for Innovation and Creativity at Work. In C. Ford (ed.), *Handbook of Organisational Creativity* (pp.211–237). London: Taylor & Francis.

Thank you for reading this book.